Mental Health in Your School

Mental Health in Your School

A Guide for Teachers and Others Working in Schools

Young Minds

Jessica Kingsley Publishers
London and Bristol, Pennsylvania

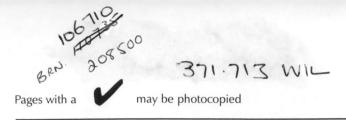

The right of Young Minds to be identified as authors of this work has
been asserted by them in accordance with the Copyright, Designs and
Patents Act 1988.
First published in the United Kingdom in 1996 by
Jessica Kingsley Publishers Ltd
116 Pentonville Road
London N1 9JB, England
and
1900 Frost Road, Suite 101
Bristol, PA 19007, U S A

Library of Congress Cataloging in Publication Data
A CIP catalogue record for this book
is available from the Library of Congress

British Library Cataloguing in Publication Data
A CIP catalogue record for this book is available from the British Library

ISBN 1-85302-407-4

Printed and Bound in Great Britain by
Athenaeum Press, Gateshead, Tyne and Wear

'Schools…play a vital part in promoting the spiritual, cultural, mental and physical development of young people'

'The emotional development of children must continue to be a concern of mainstream education'

'Pupils with Problems'
circulars from the Department
for Education 1994 (see page 43)

This book has been written by Peter Wilson, the Director of Young Minds, in consultation with a wide range of practitioners in education and mental health, many of whom are members of Young Minds. It has been funded by the Department of Health as part of the Health of the Nation initiative to improve child and adolescent mental health.

Young Minds – The National Association for Child and Family Mental Health – is the only charity in Britain working solely to raise awareness of the mental health needs of children and young people and to campaign for better services for those in need of help.

For a membership information pack and complimentary copy of the Young Minds Magazine, please contact Christopher Allman at:

> **Young Minds**
> 102-108 Clerkenwell Road
> London EC1M 5SA
> England
> tel: 0171-336 8445
> fax: 0171-336 8446

Young Minds is a registered charity and any donations in support of this vital work are welcomed.

Contents

Foreword

We all know how important school is to children. It is a place where they find out about themselves, and the world that they are growing in to; it is a place too where they meet and learn from each other and from people who are older than themselves: older children, concerned adults, and, of course, teachers. The school is a live and busy community; it is the place for children to belong to, and be part of, outside their homes.

It can be of no surprise that what goes on in school will have a significant influence on the growth of children. Their intellectual development, their knowledge, their artistic and sporting abilities, their social awareness and their self-esteem are all affected in one way or another.

It is very much the business of school to educate; to inform, train, stimulate and prepare children for later life. About this, there can be no question. What, however, is not so fully recognised is that, through the process of education, the health of children is inevitably enhanced – not just their physical health, but also their mental health. Through acknowledgment, encouragement and achievement at school children develop confidence and a capacity to adapt and meet new challenges, which are key hallmarks of mental health. Children who are mentally healthy have, by and large, the freedom to make the most of their abilities and talents; to enjoy their work and friendships.

The mental health of children depends on many factors – and the family, of course, is of fundamental importance. However, the school can also do so much for mental health – to foster the emotional well-being of children, and to be of immediate and practical help to them when problems arise.

It is because the school has such a crucial role in this respect that this book has been written: to serve as a guide for teachers and others working in schools; to highlight some of the key issues involved in the broad realm of mental health; and to stimulate, through various training exercises, further thought and understanding.

The education and the mental health of children can so often be seen as separate. Young Minds see them as closely interrelated, and this book is intended to remind us that they are very much part of the same basic process to respect and meet the wide diversity of the needs of children.

Peter Wilson
January 1996

Children's mental health: some basic facts

All children have their ups and downs and go through a range of emotions as they grow up. With the back-up of those around them, most children cope well enough. Some, however, don't do so well. Without the right conditions and support, problems may arise which can have a significant effect on a young person's future and can lead to serious difficulties in later life. Children can become unhappy at school and refuse to attend; they can have difficulty concentrating and learning; they can become irritable, naughty or disruptive; they can get into trouble, or have eating or sleeping problems. These are problems that affect children's well-being. In schools, they are usually called emotional and behavioural problems. In this book, they will be referred to as mental health problems.

The extent of such problems varies. Some are transitory and are called mild and moderate. Others persist to the point where children become distressed, confused or out of control, and when families and friends feel they cannot manage; they are described at serious or severe.

Mental health problems are relatively common in children. Between 10 and 20 per cent of children may require help at some time – that amounts to nearly two million children under the age of 16 in England and Wales.*

As many as two per cent of all children suffer from serious mental health problems. Severe mental illness, however, is rare in young children and very uncommon in young teenagers.*

Emotional and conduct disorders are found in 10 per cent of children and 20 per cent of adolescents.*

Eating disorders occur in about one per cent of 15- to 19-year-old girls.*

'About two in one hundred children under the age of twelve are depressed to the extent that they would benefit from seeing a specialist Child Psychiatrist. However, four or five in every one hundred of this age show significant distress and some of these could be described as on the edge of depression. The rate goes up with age, so that about five teenagers in one hundred are seriously depressed, and at least twice that number show significant distress. These figures apply to stable settled populations in reasonably good social circumstances. In troubled, inner-city areas with high rates of broken homes, poor community support and raised neighbourhood crime rates, the level of depression may be twice the figures we have quoted.

These figures relating to depression mean that in a secondary school in a reasonably settled area, with one thousand children on the roll, about 50 children will be depressed in any one year. In a primary school with about 400 children on the roll in an inner-city area, about eight

---

*   *Mental Illness - The Fundamental Facts* Mental Health Foundation.1993.

children will be seriously depressed, and double that number will be significantly distressed. Other children in these schools, and often quite a lot of them, will have problems such as disruptive behaviour and learning difficulties.'*

A survey of nearly 7000 children in Sheffield found that one in four primary school-age children had been bullied during the term in which the survey was carried out.**

The mental health of children is important because:

° untreated mental health problems create distress not only in the children themselves but in all those who care for them

° unresolved problems in childhood and adolescence may continue or increase in adult life

° mental health problems in children increase demands on social services, educational services and juvenile justice resources.***

Mental health problems affect many or all aspects of a child's life. All people, agencies and services in contact with children have a part to play even though the promotion, maintenance and restoration of mental health may not be their prime purpose.

Parents and carers, teachers, social workers and GPs are all involved.* Helping these children takes time, skill and patience. Therapeutic services are few and need to be expanded to meet their needs.

---

* Graham,P. and Hughes, C. (1995) *So Young, So Sad, So Listen.* London: Gaskell
** Professor Peter Smith, University of Sheffield.
*** Department of Health (1995) *Mental Health Handbook on Child and Adolescent Mental Health.* London: HMSO

1 What has mental health got to do with schools?

'What has mental health got to do with schools? Schools are places where children should learn, mental illness is for doctors...'

There are many people who agree with that statement. Anything to do with 'mental health' or 'mental illness', they say, is not to do with schools and teachers, but with hospitals and doctors.

The purpose of this book is to take another look at that view – to raise awareness of the importance of children's mental health and the central role of the school in promoting it and helping when problems arise. Its aim is to stimulate discussion and serve as a basis for training.

2   What is mental health?

It is important to understand what we mean by mental health. Mental health is often confused with mental illness, and as such quickly passed over to psychiatrists and other specialists to sort out. But, in fact, mental health is simply what it says it is. It is about the health of the *mind* – that is, the way we feel, think, perceive and make sense of the world.

When we speak about *health* we think about something positive, more than just the absence of illness. What we have in mind are ideas about strength and vitality; about parts of ourselves functioning well together – so that when we look at *mental health* we need to take into account emotional well-being; happiness, integrity and creativity; and the capacity to cope with stress and difficulty.

Mental health, in effect, refers to the capacity to live a full, productive life, as well as the flexibility to deal with its ups and downs. In children and young people, it is especially about the capacity to learn, to enjoy friendships, to meet challenges, to develop talents and capabilities.

3 Mental health and the teacher

When we take this point of view we can see that children's mental health is very much the business of all adults and friends. And the teacher, of course, is especially important – because children spend so much of their time in school and look to the teacher and other staff for support and guidance. Schools are places where children develop their intellectual capacities, as well as broaden their social and emotional potential.

The teacher plays a crucial role in providing a wide range of opportunities and possibilities to help children learn both about the outside world and themselves. Education and mental health are closely intertwined.

4 Providing a healthy culture...providing an effective school

How well a school can carry out its educational task and promote mental health depends on its values and principles, and on the general culture it manages to build and maintain. This is ultimately the responsibility of the school governors, the head teacher and senior staff. The direction that is laid down at the top sets the tone throughout the entire school.

What matters above all else is that everyone in the school is treated with *respect*. This includes the teachers, the non-teaching staff and the parents as well as the children. All can add to the development of policies and attitudes that ensure a secure environment, and build on positive strengths and good practice.

Promoting mental health in schools, then, is not just about picking up children's problems; it is about providing a healthy culture – and this in turn depends on ensuring that a school is working effectively. We know from research* that

---

* Mortimore, P. (1995) *Effective schools: Current Impact and Future Potential*. London: London Institute of Education.

schools which are effective have a number of characteristics in common:

- they all place particular emphasis on raising children's self-esteem
- they provide positive feedback
- they maintain clear and fair discipline
- they focus on the importance of achievement in the curriculum and hold high expectations of all children regardless of their particular difficulties
- they make sure they work collaboratively with people in the community, and act, as much as possible, with parental involvement.

These schools create, in other words, healthy cultures. They are places in which the mental health of children – their emotional well-being – is enhanced: children are valued and supported; their individual needs are understood and met; their difficulties are noticed and listened to; and their parents or guardians are informed and consulted.

In these schools, intimidation, racism, sexism, bullying and other forms of violence and abuse are not tolerated. When they do occur, children know problems will be dealt with, as speedily and fairly as possible. They are also taught how to cope with them. Under these conditions, children feel free to learn – they want to go to school. The foundations for sound education and mental health are set.

5 Mental health, mental illness and special educational needs

The majority of children and teenagers lead emotionally healthy lives. This does not mean that they are perfect. They struggle with all the usual difficulties and disappointments of growing up. They are affected from time to time by adverse events in their lives, such as a bereavement or loss, and they inevitably become distressed, sad and angry. These reactions are natural; they are necessary ways of adjusting to new, often difficult circumstances.

What matters is that children do not become overwhelmed by these feelings so that they get stuck and are unable to get on with their lives. Children in 'good enough' mental health are able, in fact, to learn from their difficulties and make the most of their abilities. They are curious about what is going on; interested in how they feel and making sense of the world. They want to know more about themselves, their friends, their families, their communities and beyond. They are, more or less, happy, assertive and confident, and have an awareness of what is right and wrong. And they are prepared to try out new experiences and take risks without being destructive to themselves or to others. These are the essential qualities which most people regard as making up the mental health of children, although clearly, families from different cultures and ethnic backgrounds will value certain qualities and principles more highly than others, according to their own beliefs and ways of living.

MENTAL ILLNESS

There are many others, however, who do not cope so well. Some – a small minority – may have severe emotional and psychological problems. They may be diagnosed as having a mental illness, such as clinical depression or schizophrenia. They may have extreme difficulty in making sense of the world; they may become very confused, unable to distinguish between reality and fantasy; and they may relate in an odd and bizarre way or inappropriately to other people.

Some may become very withdrawn and self-preoccupied while others become very excitable and out of control. These children require specialist help from Child and Adolescent Mental Health Services and are also likely to have special educational needs.

MENTAL HEALTH PROBLEMS

There are many children, however, who are not so incapacitated, but who nevertheless can become very distressed and have difficulty in dealing with the strains and pressures of everyday life, not to mention the demands of growing up.

These children are not 'mentally ill', but they do have significant problems – mental health problems – at different times in their lives. Many of these are quite mild and temporary and are often reactive to what is going on in families and at school. These problems are manageable with help from friends, parents and teachers, and they pass as the children move on and find new solutions.

Others, however, are more serious; they don't go away so easily and they can cause a great deal of upset to children and those who are caring for them. They are often very complex, brought on by a combination of genetic, developmental, family and social factors. Some may be particularly related to experiences children have had, or are having, in their families, such as abuse, neglect or parental violence or discord; others may be more to do with experiences outside the family, in the community or school, such as bullying or racism.

These kind of problems can build up so that children may become particularly anxious, frightened or angry, or feel undermined, discriminated against and isolated.

Children have, in other words, a wide range of mental health problems (the more severe and persistent are referred to as 'mental disorders' in child psychiatry.) Some children cover up these problems very effectively in school, and display more disturbed behaviour at home. Others, however, express them in various forms of emotional and behavioural difficulties in school, as well as in some of the learning difficulties with which teachers are familiar.

Most of these children have special educational needs that require special provision. For the majority of these children, these needs can be met within the healthy culture of an effective learning environment in a school. Teachers and other school staff are well-placed to identify difficulties as they occur, and have an important role in finding ways to help – through what they can do themselves, using help in the school and drawing on outside resources.*

---

* See page 50 for list of resources.

21

The 1993 Education Act required the Sectretary of State to issue a Code of Practice for special educational needs. This lays down a graded set of arrangements designed to provide careful assessment and intervention, in collaboration with parents. For those children who are not able to overcome their difficulties at school without a more structured framework of support, these arrangements ensure that additional help is available in conjunction with educational psychologists and other agencies, such as the local Child and Family Consultation Service and Child Psychiatry Department.

6 A child's journey...

WHAT ARE THE PRESSURES THAT EVERY CHILD HAS TO CONTEND WITH IN GOING TO SCHOOL AND GROWING UP?

Life will be challenging to children at all stages of development as they go through school. Times of transition, tackling new subjects, joining new groups, having new teachers, preparing for public examinations – all are critical points in a child's life. They open up new possibilities of learning, but equally they present difficulties and pressures which, for some, can be very difficult to handle.

The way in which a child copes with these situations, and is helped to deal with them by friends, family and teachers, can have a major bearing on his or her mental health. Some children will approach these challenges and changes with more confidence than others, and with varying degrees of assistance from other people.

FROM HOME TO PRIMARY SCHOOL

The most dramatic change of all is the first move from everyday family life at home to daily life at school. Most children are excited by this experience and are ready to enter into new relationships and make the most of the opportunities that are available. Others, however, are more timid, afraid of losing the familiar protection of their parents, and overawed by all the new children and adults and the boisterousness of the playground. They may become frightened of going to school, and their parents, too, may find it difficult letting them go. Others may not be able to concentrate and learn or they may deal with their uncertainty by becoming disruptive and aggressive.

Nursery school can help with this crucial first transition, providing young children with the chance of getting to know children and adults outside the family, introducing new activities and developing language and social skills.

It is especially important to notice signs of difficulty at this stage (see page 28) – not only to help children settle at school, but also to lay the basis for a positive attitude throughout their schooldays.

PRIMARY SCHOOL

The years that children spend at primary school are of crucial importance for their intellectual, social and emotional growth, and the development of their self-esteem. Primary school offers children the opportunity to establish their own independence from home and to discover all sorts of things about themselves and the outside world beyond their family. They learn about making relationships, and they develop new ways of thinking. They benefit especially from the demands of the curriculum, adapting to the more objective disciplines of science and mathematics and acquiring new factual knowledge.

Children in primary school need above all a reliable and consistent structure to their day in which to feel secure and learn most effectively. Provided they are well-prepared, most children respond positively to new experiences. They are curious and ready to develop their capacity to learn. They are interested in exploring their differences and stimulated by the new competitive challenges. Sudden changes of routine, however, or unexpected activities, can be unsettling for some, at least in the beginning. Teachers and other staff can make a great difference to these children by allowing them time to adjust and by explaining clearly what is being planned.

THE TRANSITION FROM PRIMARY SCHOOL TO SECONDARY SCHOOL

The move from primary to secondary school is a major change in a young person's life. It represents one of the most significant steps in growing up and achieving greater maturity. Like the earlier move into primary school, it entails the loss of all that has been familiar: teachers, routines, sometimes friends. It is a transition to a different, much larger environment – from feeling big to feeling small – with more people, more strangers and new rules and procedures. The more complex organisation of the secondary school requires a child to move from one class to another and from one group to another. Children can no longer rely upon having the same physical place to belong in, or the same children in the classroom with them. They must also adapt to working with different teachers and to more tests and exams.

Again, most young people react positively to the new regime, but many feel quite overwhelmed. Some children panic and refuse to go to school at this point in their school lives. Teachers and other staff need to be attentive to signs of stress, both in the last term of primary school when children are anticipating the loss of their familiar life and in the first year of secondary school after the transition has taken place.

Good communication between teachers in primary and secondary schools can assist children through this transition; transferring records before secondary school starts, for example, can be useful. It can also help to ask the children themselves to suggest ways of getting used to the new school, or arrange a day visit in the term before starting at the new school.

SECONDARY SCHOOL

Secondary school life is a testing time for young people. Academically, socially and emotionally, all may have difficulty in balancing and dealing with the demands of the curriculum, the pressures of group living and the adolescent tasks of growing up. Teenagers have their own particular problems, not least in coming to terms with the bodily changes of puberty, and establishing a separate identity and independence from parents.

Adolescence is also a time of questioning authority, challenging assumptions and testing limits. These are major preoccupations that can well take young people's minds away from concentrating on their work at different times. Most handle these tensions well enough so they can enjoy the new experiences and still get on with their work. Others, however, may become too wrapped up in these changes or frightened by them; they may lose themselves in the excitement of it all or become rigid and controlling. Either way, mental health problems can develop, and school work is likely to suffer.

Of increasing concern for most young people in the later years of secondary school are the questions of whether or not – and in what ways – they are going to achieve, and what they are going to do once they have left school. Many feel under considerable pressure to succeed at school and to pass exams, and some have to struggle to meet high parental expectations. The fear of failure can be very troubling and for some quite intolerable. They may push themselves too hard and worry excessively, or they may give up and pull out altogether. Some may feel school to be irrelevant to their 'real' lives in the outside world, or, for example, in some areas especially, to the problems of unemployment.

The teacher is in a good position to keep an eye on such strains and to offer help or reassurance, and put things in context. The teacher can tune into the anxieties young people have about their future and offer as much information and advice as possible to help them prepare. He or she can also help many young people who feel too despondent and disaffected to take a more positive attitude to the challenges ahead.

However, within the complex structure of the secondary school, it can be hard to spot problems, and difficult to keep track in a busy timetable. How do you look out for a child in one of several teaching groups, when you only see him or her twice a week? Well-established pastoral care and tutorial systems are essential to ensure adequate procedures for monitoring children who give concern, and for ensuring that problems are not overlooked.

7   Signs to look for...

WHAT DO YOU NEED TO BE ALERT TO WHEN CONSIDERING THE MENTAL HEALTH PROBLEMS OF YOUNG PEOPLE?

Children have different ways of managing the challenges and stresses of their development and school life. Much will depend on their own personal resources, their family circumstances, and the social, economic, cultural and ethnic backgrounds of the neighbourhoods and communities of which their schools are a part. Although there are some basic qualities which most people would agree constitute positive mental health in children (see page 15), it is important to bear in mind that it is very difficult to define one clear 'normal' developmental pathway through childhood and adolescence. Care always needs to be taken to understand and respect the different values of children and families from different backgrounds. Eye contact with an adult, for example, may show disrespect in some cultures, but not meeting someone's eyes may be regarded as a sign of evasiveness by others.

All children, of course, become preoccupied and worried from time to time, with problems at home or at school. They may be moody and irritable, their eating and sleeping may be affected, and they may not always have their minds on their work. There are no children who behave correctly and properly all the time. Inevitably they make mistakes and get into difficulties. Teenagers, in particular, can be remarkably unpredictable and at times rebellious, some becoming isolated within themselves while others become aggressive and intrusive.

All of this is part of growing up, and it is important to keep some perspective of what can reasonably be called 'normal development'. It is sometimes best to leave well enough alone, allowing the child the time and opportunity to find his or her own way forward. However, teachers do need to be alert to when problems *persist*, or interfere *significantly* with development and learning. The earlier children's difficulties can be identified and dealt with, the greater the chance of preventing larger problems later on.

Some children express themselves well enough through talking; others may prefer writing or artwork. Many children, however, most effectively communicate what is on their minds through their behaviour and attitude, and in the way they relate to each other. Here is a list of the major signs of possible difficulty. Different children with different kinds of problems will show a specific range of these signs.

Sudden changes in behaviour, mood or appearance
- Standard of work dropping dramatically.
- Becoming subdued or over-excited.
- Failing to hand in homework.
- Refusing to go to school.
- Dressing in a noticeably different style: looking untidy or becoming excessively concerned with cleanliness.

General behaviour

- ° Hyperactive, attention-seeking, anxious or restless.
- ° Aggressive, defiant and disruptive of others' work.
- ° Unusually quiet and passive; not in touch with what is going on; withdrawn.
- ° Odd or regressive behaviour; behaving younger than real age.
- ° Appearing tense or unhappy; showing hostility.
- ° Obsessive (e.g. overly tidy, so that little work is done).
- ° Extremely conscientious, perfectionist, "too good" (e.g. destroying their work because it is not good enough).

Pattern of work

- ° Having difficulty in settling to any piece of work and in concentrating in class.
- ° Losing enthusiasm and motivation.
- ° Becoming overly absorbed in study.

Pattern of attendance

- ° Reluctance to leave school or class.
- ° Arriving very early or late every morning.
- ° Missing school or lessons, playing truant.

Relationships

- ° Having difficulty getting on with other children in the class; having few or no friends.

Relationships

- Having difficulty getting on with other children in the class; having few or no friends.
- Being bullied or bullying others.

Younger children particularly

- Extremely clinging or demanding of a teacher; frequently breaking down in tears.
- Constantly getting into fights with other children and having temper tantrums.
- Damaging other children's work.
- Insisting on initiating sexual play.
- Being very bossy and over-organising others.

Older children particularly

- Looking unhappy and solitary, tired or unwell.
- Becoming careless or indifferent about work.
- Problems with eating (e.g. throwing away packed lunches; losing or gaining weight).
- Being drawn into promiscuity, delinquency or misusing alcohol or drugs.
- Violent behaviour in playground or class.
- Breaking the law outside school.
- Self-destructive behaviour (e.g. arm cutting).

It should be borne in mind that some of these problems can also be pointers to physical or sexual abuse. Guidance to teachers about abuse is available from local authorities and teaching unions; clear policies in schools for dealing with suspected abuse cases, and an awareness of the requirement to inform the Social Services department, are essential. According to the The Children Act 1989, each school should have a designated member of staff trained in child protection. Everyone working in education should be able to recognise the various symptoms of physical and sexual abuse and neglect. (See DES 4/88, *Protection in School – a handbook for developing child protection training*, National Children's Bureau 1995.)

These signs do not automatically mean that a child has a mental health problem, but may they be indicative of one.

Key questions to ask are:

° How extreme is the behaviour or attitude?

° How prolonged or persistent is it?

° Are there sudden changes in behaviour?

° How 'driven' or out of control is the child? (N.B. this is not to say that teachers should wait until a child is out of control before seeking help.)

° Is there a marked contrast between the way a child behaves at home and at school?

° How is the behaviour affecting other members of the school community?

It is important for the teacher to keep an accurate and dated record of observations and concerns so that he or she can discuss actual events or changes in behaviour with parents or other professionals as a next step. It is also helpful to know whether a child has been offered help, or is receiving professional help, outside the school. It is particularly important to know whether a child is on medication for any reason because that may be having an effect on his or her behaviour.

There is a great deal of concern and uncertainty among many teachers about some children who cause serious disruption in the classroom and interfere with their own and other children's progress. These children are commonly called hyperactive; they are restless, inattentive, impulsive. They cannot concentrate and they find it difficult to complete assigned tasks. There are, of course, many children, especially boys, who tend to be very active physically and who are at times boisterous and unable to settle. With patience and firm structure in the classroom, however, most are able to keep within the boundaries and gradually learn to control themselves and apply themselves to what is required.

Some children, however, do not respond to such everyday management. Their hyperactive behaviour is persistent; it takes over all aspects of their lives at school and at home, and invariably leads to angry, difficult and anti-social behaviour. These children need to be referred for specialist help through the Special Needs Co-ordinator to the local Child Mental Health Service, and seen for assessment by a child psychiatrist.

They may well be diagnosed as having Attention Deficit Hyperactivity Disorder (ADHD).* This basically means that they suffer from deficits in their ability to focus their attention and control their impulsive behaviour. There is no single cause for such a disorder. In the majority of cases, both biological and environmental factors play a part and it is very important that teachers and child mental health professionals work collaboratively in assessing and developing ways of managing these children.

---

* See resources on ADHD on page 50

For some children, child psychiatrists may suggest medication to enable them to settle and concentrate enough to benefit from teaching and to take their place appropriately in the classroom without incurring the criticism and hostility which they usually arouse. The most common medication is called Ritalin, and for some children it can have a remarkably positive effect on their behaviour.

It is important to stress, however, that medication does not 'cure' the condition, nor does it provide a lasting treatment. Moreover, it should not be recommended as the first or only treatment. It should be reserved for certain children who have been carefully diagnosed, and seen as part of an overall management approach in which help is given to the family and to the child both in child mental health clinics and in the school.

In the classroom, hyperactive children and those suffering from ADHD can be helped significantly if time and sufficient attention is given to their needs. It can make a great deal of difference, for example, if such children are provided with a clear structured routine in which they are protected from distractions and intrusions. It can help to seat them near the front of the classroom with quieter children near them to help calm them.

It is important too, to give them clear instructions and allow them extra time to complete their task. Giving them work in smaller portions can help to compensate for their short attention span. Most children with ADHD often possess artistic and creative talents which can be developed, as well as any other talents they may have, to raise their self-esteem, and teachers can reward them with praise for their successes in these areas.

8 The teacher can help...

The teacher has a key role to play in contributing to the mental health of students. Clearly his or her basic task is to teach and facilitate learning – and this *in itself* will be of considerable benefit to children's sense of well-being in broadening their knowledge and level of competence. How the teacher carries out this task can make a great deal of difference to how children respond to the challenges of learning, and feel positively about themselves. It matters, for example, that the teacher:

- ° builds on children's strengths, taking care to grade the steps of teaching to make achievement possible

- ° explains patiently what children have to do and helps them to assess their own progress

- ° reassures children about making mistakes; that this is a part of learning, and not a sign of failure

- ° provides interesting and stimulating materials.

What is important in all this is that the teacher creates a secure and encouraging environment in which children feel supported enough to be receptive to what is being said to them, to express themselves and take on the risks of finding out and learning.

The teacher's attitudes to the emotional problems of children are also very important – and can affect the behaviour of classes significantly.
The teacher has considerable influence and is in a position of authority to ensure a safe atmosphere in the classroom, through establishing a firm and clear disciplinary framework in which children can concentrate and learn.

He or she can, time permitting, give the space and the opportunity to children to talk about their thoughts and feelings. These may be about difficulties in their relationships and families; they may also be about worries and questions that arise naturally from what they are learning – topics, tests or activities, that may touch on their personal and family lives.

He or she can, above all, listen.
The teacher may be the one person outside the family that some children feel they can or want to talk to about a variety of concerns – such as parents separating, a death in the family, friendship problems, physical development or sexual worries.

These preoccupations may arise in discussion in the course of lessons, particularly in some subjects such as English, PSE or Physical Education. It is important that the teacher is receptive and sensitive while remaining careful and clear both to him or herself and to the children about the limits of what he or she can do. Most children understand these limits, and within them, they appreciate being heard and having their problems taken seriously.

It can help if the teacher makes clear to the child when he or she is available to talk, and how much time he or she has. It is often sufficient simply to listen to the child, conveying sympathy or concern, and reflecting back or summarising what is on the child's mind. It may be necessary to follow up with one or two further talks, but it is generally inadvisable to go beyond this on an individual basis.

It is important to help the child share his or her problem with other people in the family or school. The teacher needs to be clear about matters of confidentiality and parental involvement, in relation, for example, to contraception and pregnancy in girls under sixteen, or to the disclosure of possible sexual abuse within the family. (See page 31)

9   Teachers need support

It is essential that the teacher is given support, particularly in relation to those children who are in persistent difficulty. Many problems can be managed in the day-to-day life of the school, but there are some which cannot be dealt with in the classroom alone, and the teacher should not be expected to act as a therapist or a social worker. When the teacher is having particular difficulties, it may be helpful for him or her to look critically at what he or she is doing and at what is happening in the school generally. However, it is important that the teacher does not see it as failure if he or she cannot handle a troubled child on his or her own. It is *always important* to talk over problems with other staff. Getting outside help for a child, too, can often be the most positive way of tackling a difficulty before it becomes a crisis.

The teacher is in a key position to notice signs of distress or disturbance. These may often be quite obvious, but in many cases it may well take time to be sure whether or not to be concerned and to take further action. Making judgements about the emotional well-being of children is rarely straightforward, and the teacher needs the opportunity to check his or her concerns with other staff.

Different schools have different arrangements to assist the teacher. The principal point of reference in most schools is a Special Needs Co-ordinator (SENCO) or Head of Year.

Some schools also provide for consultation amongst staff for managing difficult children. The Special Eduation Needs Code of Practice sets out various stages of procedure in which arrangements are made for the teachers to keep records of his or her observations of children they are concerned about, and for liaison with other colleagues both in and outside the school. There are a number of professionals who are available to the teacher, such as educational psychologists, educational welfare officers, school nurses, school doctors, child psychotherapists and child psychiatrists. Young Minds has a series of leaflets about the different services and what they do.

Access to these professionals is generally arranged through the Special Needs Co-ordinator (SENCO), or Head of Pastoral Care. It is not always necessary for a particular child to be seen by a professional outside the school; it may be sufficient for the teacher to talk about the problem with the professional. This can be a useful process of assessment and can lead to new strategies for support.

10 Working with parents and carers

Keeping in touch with and informing parents and carers of their children's progress is basic to good practice in schools and contributes significantly to the well-being of all children. Involving parents and carers of children who are having problems is especially important. Many of the difficulties which children have at school have their origins in family life.

The expectations that children have of their teachers (and the lessons) may be influenced quite strongly by their experiences of adults at home. It can help a great deal, therefore, to find ways of meeting and getting to know parents and carers from early on. Most are very concerned about their children, and when difficulties arise, there is much to be gained from listening to them and negotiating with them on how best to help their child. The sooner problems are shared between parents, carers and teachers, the greater the possibility of preventing things getting out of hand, both at home and at school.

It is particularly important to have the parents' and carers' understanding and agreement to a child being referred for professional help outside the school. Every effort needs to be made to help the child cope with juggling school and keeping appointments with the professional concerned.

11 So... what has mental health got to do with schools?

A great deal!

CHILDREN'S MENTAL HEALTH

° is basically about their well-being – emotionally, socially, educationally

° is the business of everyone – and not least teachers, who are so central in children's lives

° is promoted in healthy cultures in effective schools.

All children have their share of stress and problems; they all face the same pressures and challenges as they grow up and go through school. Most children meet them with enthusiasm and curiosity, and benefit, both educationally and emotionally, from all that school offers. However, some children – not an insignificant minority – have particular difficulties. They don't feel well or happy, they don't get on with friends or grown-ups; they are not learning to the best of their abilities. Some act out aggressively; others are quiet and withdrawn. These children are not mentally ill, but they are not enjoying positive mental health. They all have emotional and behavioural problems of one kind or another.

The teacher is in a central position to promote the mental health of his or her students, through teaching, establishing clear rules, providing encouragement and setting a good example. The teacher can also do a great deal to help those with problems through good management, offering the chance to talk, listening, noticing signs of difficulties and bringing in extra help from within and outside the school when necessary.

The 1994 Special Educational Needs Code of Practice is now in place. It lays out a clear framework of management for teachers to help those children in difficulty and to get the support they need.

The mental health of all children – those with and without problems – can be much enhanced in the school.

12 Read on...

Young Minds produce a series of leaflets for parents, teachers and other concerned adults, describing mental health services for children and their families, and some of the more common emotional problems experienced by young people:

- ° Why do young minds matter?
- ° What are Child and Family Consultation Services?
- ° How can psychologists help children?
- ° How can child psychotherapists help?
- ° How can family therapy help my family?
- ° Worried about a young person's eating problems?
- ° Children and young people get depressed too
- ° Bullying: why it matters
- ° Does someone in your family have a serious mental health problem?

All these, and other materials are available from Young Minds, 102–108 Clerkenwell Road, London EC1H 5SA. tel. 0171-336 8445

Pupils With Problems, Joint Circulars issued from Dept of Health and Dept for Education (DfE tel 0171 925 5542).

Circular DFE 8/94: Pupil Behaviour and Discipline

Circular DFE 9/94 DH LAC (94)9: the Education of Children with Emotional and Behavioural Difficulties.

Circular DFE 10/94: Exclusions from School.

Circular DFE 11/94: The Education of Children Otherwise than at School.

Circular DFE 12/94 DH LAC (94)10 HSG (94)24: The Education of Sick Children.

Circular DFE 13/94 DH LAC (94)11: The Education of Children being Looked After by Local Authorities.

So Young, So Sad, So Listen, Philip Graham and Carol Hughes, Gaskell/West London Health Promotion Agency (1995). ISBN 0-902241-80-X.

Published as part of the Royal College of Psychiatrists' Defeat Depression campaign. Helps parents, teachers and teenagers to recognise and understand depression, offers advice and help.

Child and Adolescent Mental Health, Handbook by Dept of Health, Social Services Inspectorate and Dept for Education, Available from HMSO Manchester Print Logistics Warehouse, Oldham Business Park, Broadgate, Chadderton, Oldham, Lancs OL9 OJA.

Of interest to all those in contact with children, including those who purchase and provide services.

With Health in Mind, Dr Zarrina Kurtz, Action for sick children (1992). ISBN 0 904076 10 5. Report on the mental health needs of children.

Helping Troubled Pupils in Secondary Schools, Ken Reid, Blackwell (1989), ISBN 0631162658

Looks at range of problems and possible reasons for them, both in school and outside (e.g. problems at home). Discusses school pastoral and counselling services, examines more persistent problems, what help is available when school-based help is not enough.

Running a Short-Term Activity Group – a handbook for volunteer leaders, by Katrin Fitzherbert. Available from the Pyramid Trust. tel: 0181-579 5108

Introduces the Pyramid scheme – 'effective preventive help for young children'. Simple screening procedure to help teachers identify children who might be at risk socially, educationally or emotionally, and to develop strategies to support them (includes social skills, confidence building), within therapeutic activity groups.

Emotional Growth and Learning, by Paul Greenhalgh, Routledge (1994), ISBN 0 415 101344

Winner of the TES/NASEN Special Needs award '94. Clarifies the processes in social interactions and relationships which influence emotional growth and learning, illustrated by relevant examples.

TEACHING PACKS

Turn Your School Around, by Jenny Moseley, LDA, ISBN 1855031744

Whole-school circle-time approach to the development of positive behaviour and self-esteem. Guidance on policy and practical issues; exercises for the classroom.

Skills for the Primary School Child, by Alysoun Moon (ed), Tacade, ISBN 0905954440

Whole-school approach to PSE in primary school. Originally aimed at developing positive approach to child protection. Good materials on developing self-esteem and supportive school ethos. Supplementary lesson cards also available – ISBN 0905954602 – covering growing and changing (sex education), bullying, rules and regulations, keeping safe in the community, the family.

Skills for Adolescents, by various authors, Tacade, ISBNs: Curriculum Guide 0933419155, Activities and Assignments 0933419163, Parents' Meetings 093341952X, Surprising

Years (for parents) 0933419171, Changes (for students) 093341918X.

Package of materials for developing health-related personal and social skills. For use with pupils approaching adolescence (10–14 years and 14–16 years).

Mental Health Pack – a Health Education Resource for Schools. Available from: North Manchester Health Promotion Service, Beech Mount, Harpurhey, Manchester M9 1XS.

Aimed mainly at secondary schools. Exercises for use in PSE and across the curriculum for developing awareness of and strategies for personal emotional well-being.

Mental Health Matters. Published by Northern Ireland Centre for Learning Resources, The Orchard Building, Stranmills College, Belfast, BT9 5DY (tel. 01232 664525). ISBN 1 85738 033 9.

Teaching pack with teacher's handbook, classroom activity cards/worksheets and video.

Bullying – Don't suffer in silence. Available from HMSO bookshops. Details from 0171 873 9090. Plus 25-minute INSET Video. £15 inc P&P from Dialogue, 46 Avondale Road, Wolverhampton WV OAJ.

An anti-bullying pack for schools from the Department for Education. £9.95.

13 The SEN Code of Practice and the School-Based Stages of Assessment

Following on from the Education Act 1993, the Department for Education issued a Code of Practice on the Identification and Assessment of Special Educational Needs.*

The Code 'recognises that there is a continuum of needs and of provision' and that 'provision for all children with special educational needs should be made by the most appropriate agency. In most cases this will be the child's mainstream school, working in partnership with parents; no statutory assessment will be necessary.'

'About 20 per cent of children may have some form of special educational needs at some time. For the majority of children, such needs will be met by their school...only in around 2 per cent of cases will the LEA be required to

---

* National Children's Bureau, Highlight no. 132, Code of Practice: Education Act 1993.

determine and arrange special educational provision by means of a statutory statement.'

There is a framework, or 'staged response' for this which all schools should implement, with support and advice from the Special Needs Co-ordinator, usually a designated member of staff. It consists of five stages.

The first three are based in the school, with, if necessary, help from external specialists. At Stages 4 and 5 the LEA share responsibility. It should be seen as a 'continuous and systematic cycle of planning, intervention and review within the school to enable the child to learn and progress.'

'The majority of children will not progress through all three school-based stages of assessment and provision. In most cases action taken at one stage will mean that the child will not have to move onto the next.'

The 'trigger' for Stage 1 is the registration of a concern that a child is showing signs of having special educational needs, together with the evidence for that concern, by any teacher at the school, by a parent, or by another professional, such as a health or social services worker.

WHAT ARE THE STAGES?

At Stage 1 the class or subject teacher:

- ° identifies a child's special educational needs
- ° consults the parents and child
- ° informs the Special Educational Needs Co-ordinator
- ° collects relevant information about the child
- ° keeps written records of the observations of the child's behaviour

° works closely with the child within the normal classroom context.

At Stage 2 the class or subject teacher continues the arrangements made at Stage 1, building upon the information already gained. The Special Needs Co-ordinator now takes the lead responsibility for ensuring that an Individual Education Plan (IEP) is drawn up, and for co-ordinating the child's programme, in close contact with the teachers. The teachers continue to work closely with the child and keep parents informed.

At Stage 3, if the child continues to have difficulties, specialists from outside the school will be consulted to assist in monitoring and reviewing the child's progress in the Individual Education Plan.

14 Who else can help?

There is a wide range of services and agencies to provide further help.

° Local child guidance, psychiatric and psychological services for children, young people and their families *(details available from Young Minds or from your local Health Authority/NHS Trust Information Service).*

° School nurse
education welfare officer
special educational needs co-ordinator
teachers' support
information about counselling skills
training courses
Inset training etc.
(details from your Local Education Authority).

° Health Promotions Agencies *(details from your local Health Authority/NHS Trust).*

° ACE (Advisory Centre for Education), 16 Aberdeen Studios, 22 Highbury Grove, N5 2EA. 0171–354 8313 (office), 0171–354 8321 (advice 2–5p.m. Monday to Friday). *(Information and advice on all aspects of state maintained school education.)*

° Anti-Bullying Campaign, 0171–378 1446. *Support for parents and teachers, fact sheets and guidelines.*

° Carlton TV, PO Box 101, London WC2N 4AW. *Send SAE (Labelled "ADD Factsheet") for comprehensive factsheet on Attention Deficit Hyperactivity Disorder.*

- Countering Bullying Unit, Professional Development Centre, Cardiff Institute of Higher Education, Cyncoed Road, Cardiff CF2 6XD. Tel 01222–506781 (a.m. only). *In-service staff development, workshops for pupils, parents, professionals.*

- FAETT (Forum for the Advancement of Educational Therapy and Therapeutic Teaching), 0181–998 4224.

- Kidscape, 152 Buckingham Palace Road, London SW1W 9TR. Tel 0171–730 3300. *Information, booklets, training packs, courses etc. on bullying.*

- MIND, the National Association for Mental Health, Granta House, 15-19 Broadway, E15 4BQ. 0181–519 2122. *Information, publications and support.*

- NASEN (National Association for Special Educational Needs), York House, Wheelwright Lane, Coventry, West Midlands CV7 9HP. *Promotes the development of children with special educational needs, and supports those who work with them.*

- National Association for Pastoral Care in Education, c/o Education Department, University of Warwick, Westwood, Coventry CV4 7AL. 01203–523810.

- National Confederation of Parent-Teacher Associations, 2 Ebbsfleet Industrial Estate, Stonebridge Rd, Gravesend, Kent DA11 9DZ. 01474–560618.

- Network '81, 1-7 Woodfield Terrace, Stanstead, Essex CM24 8AJ. *Information and guidance on the 1993 Education Act part III.*

- Youth Access, Ashby House, 62a Ashby Road, Loughborough, Leicester LE11 3AE. 01509–219420. *A national network of informal youth counselling information and advice services.*

- Youth Services/Resources. *Details from your local authority.*

15 Some training exercises

Here are some questions and examples to stimulate discussion about the key issues raised in this book. They are intended to open up thinking about the nature of mental health and the contribution that schools can make to promoting it and helping when problems arise.

Section A poses some general questions aimed at clarifying definitions of words and phrases most commonly used. They are designed to assist a general brainstorming in a group context to identify and differentiate basic assumptions and values.

Section B gives a number of brief pictures of different kinds of children and their behaviour. They are examples drawn from everyday school life and you are invited to imagine them, link them in your mind with children whom you know and are similar, and discuss how you understand and evaluate their behaviour and attitude. In thinking about them, use your experience, your knowledge of your school's structure and special educational needs policy, and the local resources in your area.

There are three sets of examples – one each for different age groups.

Section A: What is a mentally healthy child?

1. Are you clear about what 'mental health' means?

2. To what extent is the meaning of mental health influenced by social and cultural factors? Give examples.

3. To what extent is mental health influenced by 'internal' factors such as genetic, developmental or family; and by 'external' factors such as bullying, racist or sexist attitudes?

4. What comes to mind when you think of the words:

mental	happy
health	mature
ill health	adolescence
illness	regressed
disorder	violent
child protection	

5. What is the connection, in your view, between these ideas and children with emotional and behavioural problems, and with children with special educational needs?

6. Describe three children (whom you know), at different ages (say between four and eight, eight and eleven and eleven and sixteen) who you believe are leading mentally healthy lives.

   What are the key characteristics of these children?

7. How do you help a child who doesn't have these characteristics? Through education? Therapy? Treatment? How do you understand these terms?

Section B: Three sets of examples

Choose the set most relevant to you and consider the following questions:

1. How do you understand the predicament of these children?

2. Do you think they have a mental health problem?

3. What are the main factors that need to be considered?

4. What further information would you like to have to be more clear about what to do next?

5. Should you ignore the situation, or leave it for the time being to see how things develop?

6. If you think you should do something, what would your next step be?

☐ Ask the child if he or she would like to have an informal chat with you, another teacher or other member of school staff?

☐ Make sure you find a way of talking to the child's parents, to see if there is a problem at home?

☐ Talk to another member of staff, or Special Needs Co-ordinator, or Head Teacher?

☐ Insist that the child is referred to the Child and Adolescent Services?

☐ Anything else?

7. If you were drawing up an Individual Education Plan (for Stages 2 and 3 of the SEN Code of Practice), what would be your objectives?

Example set for age group 8–11

No. 1

Arthur and Bill, twins aged 9, have just been put into separate classes. Arthur is popular and seems to be progressing satisfactorily. Bill is withdrawn and has trouble reading. At break, Bill rushes up to Arthur and is distressed when he has to leave him.

No. 2

Anjum, a 10-year-old girl, makes you, her new teacher, somehow feel uncomfortable. She whines a lot, refuses to co-operate and sometimes scribbles all over the work she has just completed. She has never had a male teacher before and always seems to want your attention.

No. 3

Eleven-year-old Dean has suddenly grown into a big, tall young man. He has always been reasonably co-operative but has become surly and aggressive. He arrives late for lessons with no apology or explanation, and has started to bully smaller children. He is mixing with older boys outside school.

No. 4

Charlotte is 8. She is a friendly little girl who has always needed a bit of extra help. Her reading ability is very low, however, and because of this she needs more help with her other classwork. Some children call her 'Dumbo' and say she should go to special school.

No. 5

Wayne is an 11-year-old. He is the smallest child in the class and sometimes he is teased. This doesn't seem to bother him. He busily gets on with his work, whistles and hums tunes all the time, and occasionally talks to himself. In many ways, he is a funny little boy – he seems happy enough, yet he doesn't really have any friends and he is often seen alone in the playground. His sisters are both grown up and have left home.

No. 6

The whole class seems very restless. There is a small group of children who are kicking a ball about, banging their desks, and deliberately pushing into other children. One boy looks frightened; he's smiling all the time, standing by the door, wanting to be excused. Another child, a girl, who is usually a cheerful soul, looks sullen and is silently scribbling all over her notebook.

Example set for age group 11–16

No. 1

Anne, aged 13, has always been a keen, interested pupil who contributed in class and produced a reasonably high quality of work. Lately, however, she has become rather sullen and withdrawn and her work is handed in late and contains no original thought and hardly any effort. In one essay she wrote of wanting to kill herself.

No. 2

Ben, a boy of 15, has recently been in some minor trouble with his particular group of friends, but there seems no serious cause for concern. His mother, however, has been to see his Head of Year a number of times regarding his difficult, aggressive behaviour at home and his surly attitude.

No. 3

Sung-ah, a 16-year-old girl, has always been keen on sport. Now she spends every lunchtime running. She also has ballet lessons on Saturday mornings and a paper round on Sundays. She looks rather pale to you, and has lost weight lately.

No. 4

Dwaine is nearly 12. He arrived at this school with good reports from his previous school. However, he is dull and lethargic, sits alone in the playground and has recently been absent a number of times. His dad, apparently, has left home recently.

No. 5

Judi is a 16-year-old. She is very bright, always on the alert, and at times quite assertive and pushy. She can be provocative with the teachers, especially men, but for the most part this is manageable and she is well-liked. The standard of her academic work is high. In the last two months, she has become slightly more irritable. She looks unhappy and you have noticed that her arms are always covered.

No. 6

Recently, some of the pupils have been demonstrating their growing interest in sex. Much of the ribaldry and crude or sexist comments which are bandied about are taken in good part, but some remarks are rather 'near the mark'. One or two pupils have become upset, and two boys and two girls have not attended school for the last week, after the teacher discovered some offensive graffiti in the playground.